The Pescatarian Cookbook

Nourish Your Body and Eat Well without Skimping on Flavor with Easy and Healthy Pescatarian Recipes

The Inspirational Chef

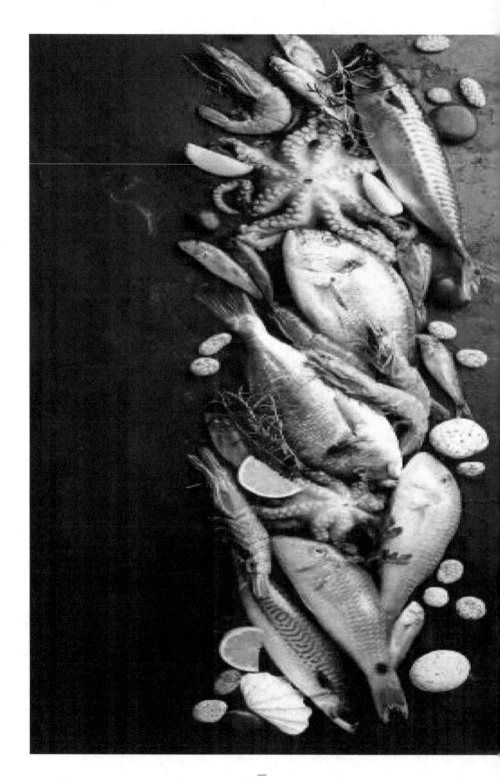

Table of Contents

Introduction

In recent times, a lot of attention has been drawn to sustainability and preserving the earth. Global population growth and increased life expectancy mean there are growing concerns about how to feed the world's population. In response to this, growth boosters are being used for animal production and preservatives used to maintain plant foods. This has led to an increase in heart disease, diabetes, and cancer. This new reality has caused a lot of the world's population to seek ways to eat healthy while preserving the planet. For some, it is switching to veganism, for others it is pescatarianism.

The word 'pescatarian' was created in the early 1990s. It is a combination of the Italian word for fish – *pesce* – and vegetarian. A pescatarian is anyone who eats a plant-based diet, along with fish and seafood. A pescatarian may also eat dairy products and eggs. They do not, however, eat any form of animal meat. A pescatarian still gets the bulk of his or her food from plant sources such as whole grains, legumes, nuts, fruits, and vegetables. They are usually people who want all the great benefits of a plant-based diet, as well as the healthy nutrients from fish.

You might be wondering whether eating fish and seafood negates the aim of vegetarianism. The answer is, not entirely. Pescatarians usually forgo meat in their diet for environmental and ethical reasons, just as a vegetarian would. And they get similar results too. A pescatarian diet is helpful for weight loss and a healthy lifestyle, as studies have shown.

Fish contains omega-3 fatty acid, high-quality protein, and low fat. It is a much better source of protein than meat. A fish diet such as the Mediterranean diet or the Atkins diet has been linked to a reduced rate of heart disease, stroke and ultimately death from these diseases. Fish is also rich in vitamin B2 (riboflavin), and vitamin D, provides minerals like phosphorus and calcium, and offers variety in taste and recipes! In addition, it is essential for pregnant women as it aids the development of fetal vision and the nervous system. Its benefits for adults also include brain health.

But it is not all Kumbaya when it comes to eating fish and seafood as they can be contaminated. Some fish high in mercury include shark, tilefish, and swordfish, and these should be avoided. Larger fish tend to have more mercury than smaller ones.

In this book, we have avoided all fish that tend to contain mercury and are going to discuss ways to make fish into delicious meals. But first, let us look in more detail at some of the reasons people opt for pescatarianism:

Health Factors

A plant-based diet with fish and seafood included offers a large variety of nutrients and options. Save for some legumes and nuts, a plant-based diet has more carbs than protein and getting one's protein requirement means consuming a large portion of these protein plants.

This can be quite exhausting. But with a pescatarian diet, you get healthy nutrients from grains, fruits, and legumes as well as lean protein from fish.

Environmental factors

According to a report by the UN, raising livestock increases the earth's carbon emissions by as much as 15%. Seafood, on the other hand, has a much lower carbon footprint than livestock. Studies carried out in 2014 have shown that people who eat seafood create 46% less greenhouse gas emissions than meat eaters. It also showed that producing cheese and animal meat has a higher carbon footprint than the production of seafood.

Ethical reasons

A lot of people who think of going vegan for ethical reasons but do not think they can get all their protein from plant sources settle for pescatarianism. Some of these ethical reasons could be the inhumane and crude way some slaughterhouses kill the animals, or generally being against the killing of animals. Sometimes they are opposed to the conditions under which these animals are raised. Another ethical reason could be the poor working conditions of slaughterhouse workers.

Some pescatarians also believe it is a waste of land and resources to raise grains for the feeding of livestock when there is so much hunger in the world. Are fish not caught under the same inhumane conditions you may ask?

The answer is, not really. The aquaculture and fishing industries have taken steps to ensure fish are raised and caught in the most humane way possible. In Alaska, for example, fishing companies ensure there is no disruption in the fish population by ensuring only adult males are caught.

Benefits of a pescatarian diet

The benefits of a pescatarian diet are immense. It is a combination of the benefits of a plant-based diet and seafood, a balanced diet plan. A pescatarian diet answers the concerns some people might have about getting the required nutrients from just plant sources. Seafood is rich in B vitamins, especially vitamins B12, zinc, calcium and protein, nutrients that are hard to get from a plant-based diet.

Omega-3 fatty acid

Fish is famous for its omega-3 fatty acid. Although some plant food sources such as walnut and flaxseed contain a type of omega-3 fat, alpha-linolenic acid (ALA), it is not easily convertible by the body into eicosapentaenoic acid (EPA) and docosahexaenoic acid (DHA) which are great for the heart, the brain and one's mood. Fish such as salmon and sardines on the other hand contain both EPA and DHA.

Boost's protein intake

Getting lean protein from plant sources is not so easy as it usually comes with carbs, and to get the required amount of protein, one must eat a large portion of food.

As humans, we need about 0.8 grams of protein for every kilogram of our body weight. That means a person who is 50kg will need 40 grams of protein daily. Some people like to eat more protein than the required amount. Getting this protein from plant sources is hard, especially if you do not want extra carbs.

Thankfully, fish and other seafood are packed with lean protein. Whitefish such as cod, halibut, flounder, or haddock contain 18 grams of protein in every ounce (28). Shrimp on the other hand delivers 12 grams of protein in every 3 ounces while tuna delivers 25 grams of protein in the same. Tilapia, a popular and inexpensive fish, contains 23 grams of protein in every 3 ounces.

The great part about fish is that they are very filling, so you do not need to eat a lot to get satisfied.

Access to more nutrients

It is not just lean protein you get from a fish diet. You also get a lot of other nutrients. Some seafood such as oysters are very high in vitamin B12, selenium and zinc. This is so high that one oyster gives about 130% of the RDI for vitamin B12 and 55% of the RDI for zinc and selenium. Shrimps are rich in choline, niacin, zinc, selenium, and vitamins E, B6 and B12. They are also high in astaxanthin, an antioxidant that reduces oxidative and inflammatory damage. Mussels contain high quantities of vitamin B12 and the other B vitamins as well as selenium and manganese.

Access to more food options

Every vegetarian knows the diet can be quite limiting, and eating in regular restaurants can be a hassle, as the best you can get in most cases is cheesy pasta. But with a pescatarian diet, you will have access to oysters, shrimp and fish which can be grilled, sautéed, and baked.

Reduces the chance of heart disease

Fish and seafood contain omega-3 fatty acid which is great for the heart. There is strong evidence that eating fish and taking fish oil is good for the heart. They are so good that they get a nod from the American Heart Association, which recommends eating fish at least twice a week. How does fish work for the heart? Fish contains omega-3 fatty acid which reduces inflammation in the body. This also includes inflammation that can damage the blood vessels and lead to stroke and other heart diseases.

Omega-3 fatty acids benefit the heart by decreasing triglycerides, slightly lowering blood pressure, reducing irregular heartbeats, and reducing blood clotting. Fish high in omega-3 fatty acids include Atlantic mackerel, cod, herring, lake trout, salmon, sardines, and tuna. However, tuna contains some amount of mercury. Although this is countered by its high selenium content, tuna should be eaten in moderation.

How to shop and store seafood

Now that we have established that seafood is great for you, how do you shop for and store it? Fish, unlike plant foods, is highly perishable and improper storage can taint its taste. The first thing to know is that fish and seafood have a short shelf life so you will have to shop for them quite frequently.

Here are a few things to take into consideration when buying fish and seafood:

When shopping for fish and seafood in a supermarket, look out for the Marine Stewardship Council (MSC) sticker. The sticker indicates that the fish has come from sustainable fisheries and your purchase will be helping the environment.

Eat a variety of fish. There is already a large demand for certain fish species such as Atlantic cod and salmon, and these are therefore overfished. Going with other fish varieties will be helpful to both your pocket and the environment. Anchovies, abalone clams, crayfish, hake, farmed mussels and oysters are all tasty sustainable choices.
Buy local. If possible, buy fish caught by your local fisheries. This means they are fresh and have not travelled from halfway across the world to your supermarket.

When shopping, buy your fish and seafood just before you leave the supermarket. This way they do not stay out of the fridge or freezer for too long.

Keep your fish and seafood bloodless and in the coldest part of your freezer or refrigerator. Jot down the date each was kept in the freezer, so it does not stay in there too long and lose its taste. It is not ideal to freeze fish for more than 3 months, and prawns and shrimps for more than 6 months. Also take into consideration the time it spent in the supermarket before your purchase.

Now that you are well caught up on the fundamentals of the pescatarian diet, let us dig in to some healthy and yummy recipes.

10-Day Meal Plan

Day	Breakfast	Lunch	Dinner
Monday	Vanilla Steel-cut Oatmeal	Spaghetti Squash Primavera	Moroccan stir fry
Tuesday	Slow Cooker Butternut Squash Oatmeal	Tofu Tikka Masala	Asian kebabs
Wednesday	Fruit Salad with Lemon Ginger Syrup	Avocado Toast with Herbs and Peas	Chickpea stew
Thursday	Banana Pancakes	Stuffed Sweet Potatoes	Butternut squash salad
Friday	Classic French Toast	Hawaiian Burger	Enchilada casserole
Saturday	Oatmeal Muffins	Mediterranean Rice	Quinoa salad
Sunday	Omelet with Chickpea Flour	Harissa Bulgur Bowl	Mediterranean budda bowl
Monday	Carrot Cake Oatmeal	Chipotle Cilantro Rice	Avocado salad
Tuesday	Grilled Cauliflower Wedges	Haddock Pie	Vegan curry
Wednesday	Oatmeal and Peanut Butter Breakfast Bar	Oat-Crusted Fried Herring	Brussels sprouts

Breakfast

Vanilla Steel-Cut Oatmeal

Preparation Time: 5 Minutes
Cooking Time: 40 minutes
Servings: 4

Ingredients

- 4 cups water
- Pinch sea salt (optional)
- 1 cup steel-cut oats
- ¾ cup unsweetened almond milk
- 2 teaspoons pure vanilla extract

Instructions

1. Place the water and salt (if desired) into a large pot over high heat and bring to a boil.
2. Reduce the heat to low and stir in the oats. Cook for about 30 minutes until the oats are soften, stirring occasionally.
3. Add the milk and vanilla and stir well. Cook for about 10 minutes more until your desired consistency is reached.
4. Remove the cereal from the heat and serve warm.

Nutrition Information

Calories: 187; Fat: 0g; Protein: 9.2g; Carbohydrates: 28.8g

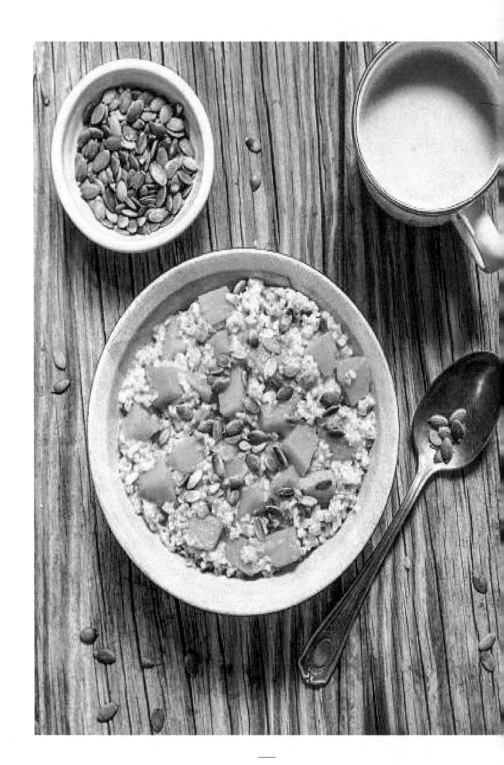

Slow Cooker Butternut Squash Oatmeal

Preparation Time: 15 Minutes
Cooking Time: 6-8 hours
Servings: 4
Ingredients

- 1 cup steel-cut oats

- 3 cups water

- 2 cups cubed (½-inch pieces) peeled butternut squash

- ¼ cup unsweetened coconut milk

- 1 tablespoon chia seeds

- 1½ teaspoons ground ginger

- 2 teaspoons yellow (mellow) miso paste

- 1 tablespoon sesame seeds, toasted

- 1 tablespoon chopped scallion, green parts only

Instructions

1. Mix together the oats, water, and butternut squash in a slow cooker.
2. Cover and cook on Low for 6 to 8 hours, or until the squash is tender when tested with a fork. Mash the cooked butternut squash with a potato masher or heavy spoon. Stir together the butternut squash and oats until well mixed.
3. Mix together the milk, chia seeds, ginger, and miso paste in a small bowl and stir to combine. Add this mixture to the squash mixture and stir well.
4. Ladle the oatmeal into bowls and serve hot topped with sesame seeds and scallion.

Nutrition Information

Calories: 229; Fat: 4.9g Carbohydrates: 39.7g; Protein: 7.1g

Banana Pancakes

Preparation Time: 5 Minutes

Cooking Time: 15 Minutes

Servings: 4

Ingredients

- 2 tablespoons ground flaxseeds
- 1/2 cup oat flour
- 1/2 cup coconut flour
- 1/2 cup instant oats
- 1 teaspoon baking powder
- 1/4 teaspoon kosher salt
- 1/4 teaspoon ground cardamom
- 1/4 teaspoon ground cinnamon
- 1/2 teaspoon coconut extract
- 1 cup banana
- 2 tablespoons coconut oil, at room temperature

Instructions

1. To make the "flax" egg, in a small mixing dish, whisk 2 tablespoons of the ground flaxseeds with 4 tablespoons of the water. Let it sit for at least 15 minutes.

2. In a mixing bowl, thoroughly combine the flour, oats, baking powder and spices. Add in the flax egg and mashed banana. Mix until everything is well incorporated.

3. Heat 1/2 tablespoon of the coconut oil in a frying pan over medium-low flame. Spoon about 1/4 cup of the batter into the frying pan; fry your pancake for approximately 3 minutes per side.

4. Repeat until you run out of batter. Serve with your favorite fixings and enjoy!

Nutrition Information

Calories: 302; Protein: 7.1g; Carbohydrates: 37.2g; Fats: 15g

Classic French Toast

Preparation Time: 5 Minutes
Cooking Time: 15 Minutes
Servings: 2
Ingredients

- 1 tablespoon ground flax seeds
- 1 cup coconut milk
- 1/2 teaspoon vanilla paste
- A pinch of sea salt
- A pinch of grated nutmeg
- 1/2 teaspoon ground cinnamon
- 1/4 teaspoon ground cloves
- 1 tablespoon agave syrup
- 4 slices bread

Instructions

1. In a mixing bowl, thoroughly combine the flax seeds, coconut milk, vanilla, salt, nutmeg, cinnamon, cloves, and agave syrup.
2. Dredge each slice of bread into the milk mixture until well coated on all sides.
3. Preheat an electric griddle to medium heat and lightly oil it with a nonstick cooking spray.
4. Cook each slice of bread on the preheated griddle for about 3 minutes per side until golden brown.

Nutrition Information

Calories: 233; Fats: 6.5g; Carbohydrates: 35.5g; Protein: 8.2g

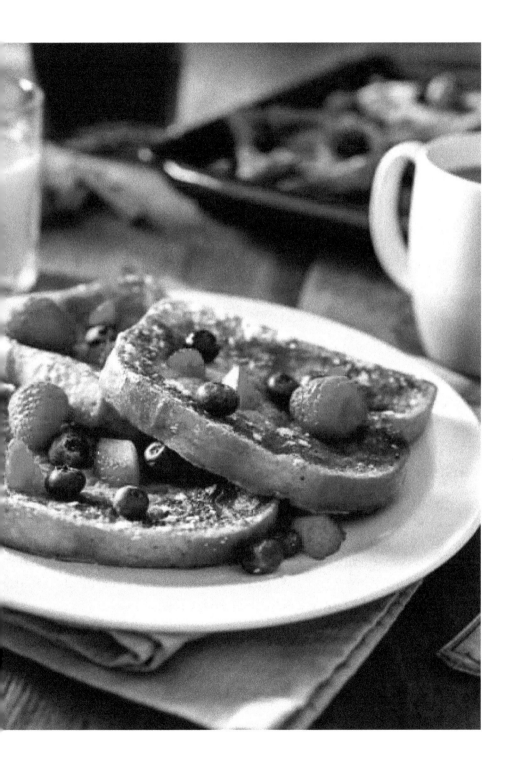

Oatmeal Muffins

Preparation Time: 10 Minutes
Cooking Time: 20 Minutes
Servings: 12
Ingredients

- ½ cup of hot water
- ½ cup of raisins
- ¼ cup of ground flaxseed
- 2 cups of rolled oats
- ¼ teaspoon of sea salt
- ½ cup of walnuts
- ¼ teaspoon of baking soda
- 1 banana
- 2 tablespoons of cinnamon
- ¼ cup of maple syrup

Instructions

1. Whisk the flaxseed with water and allow the mixture to sit for about 5 minutes.
2. In a food processor, blend all the ingredients along with the flaxseed mix. Blend everything for 30 seconds, but do not create a smooth substance. To create rough-textured cookies, you need to have a semi-coarse batter.
3. Put the batter in cupcake liners and place them in a muffin tin. As this is an oil-free recipe, you will need cupcake liners. Bake everything for about 20 minutes at 350 degrees.
4. Enjoy the freshly made cookies with a glass of warm milk.

Nutrition Information

Calories: 133; Fat: 2g; Carbohydrates: 27g; Protein: 3g

Carrot Cake Oatmeal

Preparation Time: 10 Minutes

Cooking Time: 10 Minutes

Servings: 1

Ingredients

- 1 cup, water
- ½ teaspoon, cinnamon
- 1 cup, rolled oats
- Salt
- ¼ cup, raisins
- ½ cup, shredded carrots
- 1 cup, non-dairy milk
- ¼ teaspoon, allspice
- ½ teaspoon, vanilla extract

Toppings:
- ¼ cup, chopped walnuts
- 2 tablespoons, maple syrup
- 2 tablespoons, shredded coconut

Instructions

1. Put a small pot on low heat and bring the non-dairy milk, oats, and water to a simmer.

2. Now, add the carrots, vanilla extract, raisins, salt, cinnamon, and allspice. You need to simmer all of the ingredients, but do not forget to stir them. You will know that they are ready when the liquid is fully absorbed into all of the ingredients (in about 7-10 minutes).

3. Transfer the thickened dish to bowls. You can drizzle some maple syrup on top or top them with coconut or walnuts.

Nutrition Information

Calories: 210; Fat: 11.48g; Carbohydrates: 10.37g; Protein: 3.8g

Grilled Cauliflower Wedges

Preparation Time: 22 Minutes
Cooking Time: 40 Minutes
Servings: 4

Ingredients

- 1 huge head cauliflower
- 1 teaspoon ground turmeric
- 1/2 teaspoon squashed red pepper chips
- 2 tablespoons olive oil
- Lemon juice, extra olive oil, & pomegranate seeds, discretionary

Instructions

1. Remove leaves and trim originate from cauliflower. Cut cauliflower into eight wedges. Blend turmeric and pepper pieces. Brush wedges with oil; sprinkle with turmeric blend.
2. Grill, secured, over medium-high warmth or cook 4 in. from heat until cauliflower is delicate, 9 minutes on each side.
3. Whenever wanted, shower with lemon juice and extra oil and present with pomegranate seeds.

Nutrition Information

Calories: 180; Fat: 9g; Carbohydrates: 10.52g; Protein: 2.1g

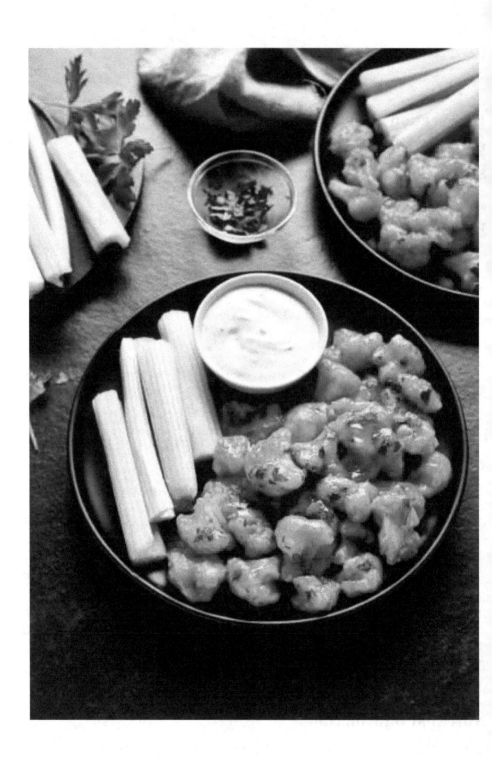

Oatmeal and Peanut Butter Breakfast Bar

Preparation Time: 10 Minutes
Cooking Time: 0 minutes
Servings: 8

Ingredients

- 1½ cups date, pit removed
- ½ cup peanut butter
- ½ cup old-fashioned rolled oats

Instructions

1. Grease and line an 8" x 8" baking tin with parchment and pop to one side.
2. Grab your food processor, add the dates and whizz until chopped.
3. Add the peanut butter and the oats and pulse.
4. Scoop into the baking tin then pop into the fridge or freezer until set.
5. Serve and enjoy.

Nutrition Information

Calories: 459; Fat: 8.9g; Carbohydrates: 98.5g; Protein: 7.7g

Lunch

Spaghetti Squash Primavera

Preparation Time: 10 Minutes

Cooking Time: 40 Minutes

Servings: 4

Ingredients

- 1 large spaghetti squash (roughly 4 pounds), halved and seeded
- 3 tablespoons extra-virgin olive oil, divided
- 1 onion, chopped
- 2 cups chopped broccoli florets
- ½ cup pitted and sliced green olives
- 1 cup halved cherry tomatoes
- 3 garlic cloves, minced
- 1½ teaspoons Italian seasoning
- ¾ teaspoon sea salt
- ½ teaspoon black pepper
- Pine nuts, for garnish (optional)
- Walnut Parmesan or store-bought vegan Parmesan, for garnish (optional)
- Red pepper flakes, for garnish (optional)

Instructions

1. Preparing the Ingredients.
2. Preheat the oven to 400°F.
3. Line a baking sheet with parchment paper.
4. Brush the rims and the insides of both squash halves with 1 tablespoon of olive oil. Place on the prepared baking sheet, cut sides down.
5. Bake
6. Bake for 35-45 minutes, until a fork can easily pierce the flesh. Set aside until cool enough to handle for 10-15 minutes.
7. While the squash is cooling, heat 1 tablespoon of olive oil in a large skillet over medium heat.
8. Add the onion and broccoli and sauté for 3 minutes, or until the onion is soft. Add the olives and tomatoes and cook for an additional 3-5 minutes, or until the broccoli is fork-tender and the tomatoes have started to wilt. Add the garlic and cook for 1 additional minute, or until fragrant.
9. Finish and Serve
10. Remove from the heat. Use a fork to gently pull the squash flesh from the skin and separate the flesh into strands. The strands wrap around the squash horizontally, so rake your fork in the same direction as the strands to make the longest spaghetti squash noodles. Toss the noodles into the skillet with the vegetables. Add 1 tablespoon of olive oil, Italian seasoning, salt, and pepper and mix well to combine. Divide among bowls and garnish with pine nuts, Parmesan, and red pepper flakes if desired.

Nutrition Information

Calories: 125; Protein: 15g; Carbohydrates: 42g; Fat: 9g

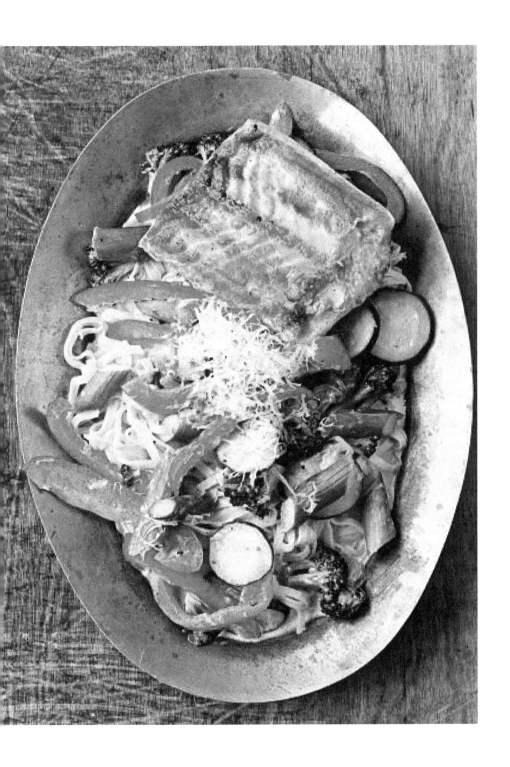

Zucchini Hummus

Preparation Time: 5 Minutes
Cooking Time: 8 Minutes
Servings: 8

Ingredients

- 1 cup diced zucchini
- 1/2 teaspoon sea salt
- 1 teaspoon minced garlic
- 2 teaspoons ground cumin
- 3 tablespoons lemon juice
- 1/3 cup tahini

Instructions

1. Place all the ingredients in a food processor and pulse for 2 minutes until smooth.
2. Tip the hummus in a bowl, drizzle with oil and serve.

Nutrition Information

Calories: 65; Fat: 5g; Carbohydrates: 3g; Protein: 2g

Tofu Tikka Masala

Preparation Time: 5 Minutes
Cooking Time: 4 Hours 10 Minutes
Servings: 4
Ingredients

- 16 ounces tofu, extra-firm, drained, ½ inch cubed
- 1 ½ teaspoon minced garlic
- 2 medium carrots, peeled sliced
- 1 medium white onion, peeled, diced
- 1 1/2 cups diced potatoes
- 1 medium red bell pepper, cored, cut into chunks
- ¾ cup frozen peas
- 2 cups cauliflower florets
- ½ tablespoon grated ginger
- ¼ teaspoon ground black pepper
- ½ teaspoon salt
- ½ teaspoon ground turmeric
- 1 ½ teaspoons cumin
- ¼ teaspoon cayenne pepper
- 1 tablespoon garam masala
- 1 teaspoon coriander
- ¼ teaspoon paprika
- ½ tablespoon maple syrup
- 15 ounces tomato sauce
- 15 ounces of coconut milk
- 2 tablespoons chopped cilantro

Instructions

1. Take a slow cooker, place all the ingredients in it, except for cilantro and peas, and stir until combined.
2. Switch on the slow cooker, shut with lid, and cook for 4 hours at a high heat setting.
3. When done, stir in peas, cook for 10 minutes, uncovering the cooker, and, when done, serve with cooked brown rice.

Nutrition Information

Calories: 303; Fat: 11.5g; Carbohydrates: 36; Protein: 15g

Queso Dip

Preparation Time: 10 Minutes
Cooking Time: 0 minutes
Servings: 6

Ingredients

- 1 cup cashews
- ½ teaspoon minced garlic
- 1/2 teaspoon salt
- 1/2 teaspoon ground cumin
- 1 teaspoon red chili powder
- 2 tablespoons nutritional yeast
- 1 tablespoon harissa
- 1 cup hot water

Instructions

1. Place all the ingredients in a food processor and pulse for 2 minutes until smooth and well combined.
2. Tip the dip in a bowl, taste to adjust seasoning and then serve.

Nutrition Information

Calories: 133; Fat: 9g; Protein: 5g; Carbohydrates: 8g

Stuffed Sweet Potatoes

Preparation Time: 15 Minutes

Cooking Time: 45 minutes

Servings: 4

Ingredients

- pounds sweet potatoes
- 1/3 cup corn kernels
- 1 cup chopped kale
- 1/4 cup diced green onion
- 3/4 cup diced tomato
- ½ teaspoon minced garlic
- 1/2 teaspoon sea salt
- 1/2 teaspoon chipotle flakes
- 1/2 teaspoon Dijon mustard
- 1/2 teaspoon smoked paprika
- 1/2 teaspoon liquid smoke
- 1/4 teaspoon ground turmeric
- 1/2 tablespoon lemon juice
- 3 tablespoons nutritional yeast
- 1/3 cup cashews, soaked, drained
- 1 1/2 cup pasta, cooked
- 1 cup baked pumpkin puree
- 1/2 cup vegetable broth

Instructions

1. Wrap each potato in a foil and then bake for 45 minutes at 375 degrees F until tender.

2. Meanwhile, prepare the cheese sauce and for this, place pumpkin and cashews in a food processor, add garlic, yeast, salt, paprika, chipotle flakes, liquid smoke, turmeric, mustard, and lemon juice, pour in broth and puree until smooth.

3. Take a pot, place it over medium-low heat, add prepared sauce, then add remaining ingredients, toss until coated, and cook for 5 minutes until kale has wilted.

4. Season the mixture with salt and black pepper, then switch heat to the low level and cook until sweet potatoes have roasted.

5. When sweet potatoes are roasted, let them stand for 10 minutes, then unwrap them, split them by slicing down the center and spoon prepared sauce generously in the center.

6. Serve straight away.

Nutrition Information

Calories: 330; Fat: 3.5g; Carbohydrates: 58g; Protein: 13g

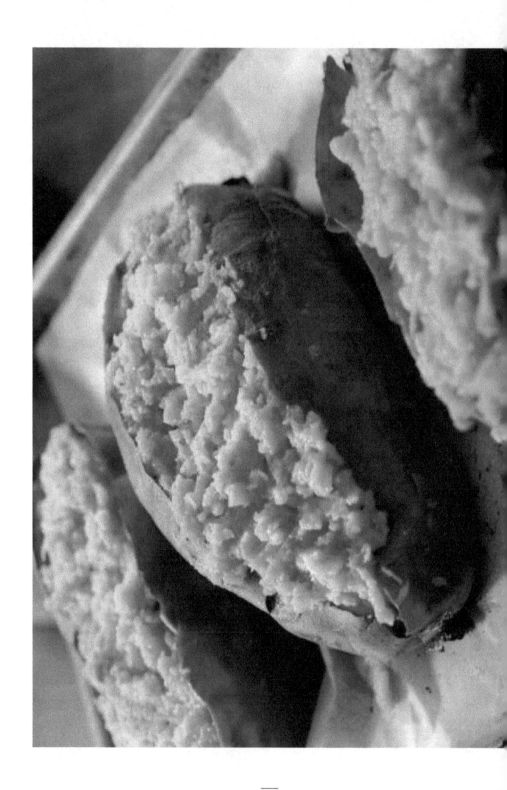

Hawaiian Burger

Preparation Time: 15 Minutes
Cooking Time: 10 Minutes
Servings: 8

Ingredients

- 3 cups cooked black beans
- 2 cups cooked brown rice
- 1 cup quick-cooking oats
- ¼ cup BBQ Sauce, plus more for serving
- ¼ cup pineapple juice
- 1 teaspoon garlic powder
- 1 teaspoon onion powder
- 1 pineapple, cut into ¼-inch-thick rings
- 8 whole-wheat buns
- Lettuce, tomato, pickles, and onion, for topping (optional)

Instructions

1. Preheat the grill to medium-high heat.

2. In a large bowl, use a fork or mixing spoon to mash the black beans.

3. Mix in the rice, oats, BBQ sauce, the pineapple juice, garlic powder, and onion powder. Continue mixing until the mixture begins to hold its shape and can be formed into patties.

4. Scoop out ½ cup of bean mixture and form it into a patty. Repeat until all of the bean mixture is used.

5. Place the patties on the hot grill and cook for 4 to 5 minutes on each side, flipping once the burgers easily release from the grill surface.

6. After you flip the burgers, place the pineapple rings on the grill, and cook for 1 to 2 minutes on each side.

7. Remove the burgers and pineapple rings from the grill. Place one patty and one pineapple ring on each bun along with a spoonful of the BBQ sauce and your favorite burger fixings and serve.

Nutrition Information

Calories: 371; Total fat: 3g; Carbohydrates: 71g; Protein: 15g

Mediterranean Rice

Preparation Time: 5 Minutes
Cooking Time: 15 Minutes
Servings: 4
Ingredients

- 3 tablespoons vegan butter, at room temperature
- 6 tablespoons scallions, chopped
- 2 cloves garlic, minced
- 1 bay leaf
- 1 thyme sprig, chopped
- 1 rosemary sprig, chopped
- 1 ½ cups white rice
- 2 cups vegetable broth
- 1 large tomato, pureed
- Sea salt and ground black pepper, to taste
- 2 ounces Kalamata olives, pitted and sliced

Instructions

1. In a saucepan, melt the vegan butter over a moderately high flame. Cook the scallions for about 2 minutes or until tender.
2. Add in the garlic, bay leaf, thyme and rosemary and continue to sauté for about 1 minute or until aromatic.
3. Add in the rice, broth, and pureed tomato. Bring to a boil; immediately turn the heat to a gentle simmer.
4. Cook for about 15 minutes or until all the liquid has absorbed. Fluff the rice with a fork, season with salt and pepper and garnish with olives; serve immediately.
5. Bon appétit!!

Nutrition Information
Calories: 403; Protein: 8.3g; Carbohydrates: 64.1g; Fats: 12g

Chipotle Cilantro Rice

Preparation Time: 15 Minutes
Cooking Time: 15 Minutes
Servings: 4

Ingredients

- 5 tablespoons olive oil
- 1 chipotle pepper, seeded and chopped
- 1 cup jasmine rice
- 1 ½ cups vegetable broth
- 1/4 cup fresh cilantro, chopped
- Sea salt and cayenne pepper, to taste

Instructions

1. In a saucepan, heat the olive oil over a moderately high flame. Add in the pepper and rice and cook for about 3 minutes or until aromatic.
2. Pour the vegetable broth into the saucepan and bring to a boil; immediately turn the heat to a gentle simmer.
3. Cook for about 18 minutes or until all the liquid has absorbed. Fluff the rice with a fork, add in the cilantro, salt, and cayenne pepper; stir to combine well. Bon appétit!

Nutrition Information

Calories: 313; Fats: 15g; Carbohydrates: 37.1g; Protein: 5.7g

Harissa Bulgur Bowl

Preparation Time: 5 Minutes
Cooking Time: 20 Minutes
Servings: 4
Ingredients

- 1 cup bulgur wheat
- 1 ½ cups vegetable broth
- 2 cups sweet corn kernels, thawed
- 1 cup canned kidney beans, drained
- 1 red onion, thinly sliced
- 1 garlic clove, minced
- Sea salt and ground black pepper, to taste
- 1/4 cup harissa paste
- 1 tablespoon lemon juice
- 1 tablespoon white vinegar
- 1/4 cup extra-virgin olive oil
- 1/4 cup fresh parsley leaves, roughly chopped

Instructions

1. In a deep saucepan, bring the bulgur wheat and vegetable broth to a simmer; let it cook, covered, for 12 to 13 minutes.
2. Let it stand for 5 to 10 minutes and fluff your bulgur with a fork.
3. Add the remaining ingredients to the cooked bulgur wheat; serve warm or at room temperature. Bon appétit!

Nutrition Information

Calories: 353; Fat: 15.5g; Carbohydrates: 48.5g; Protein: 8.4g

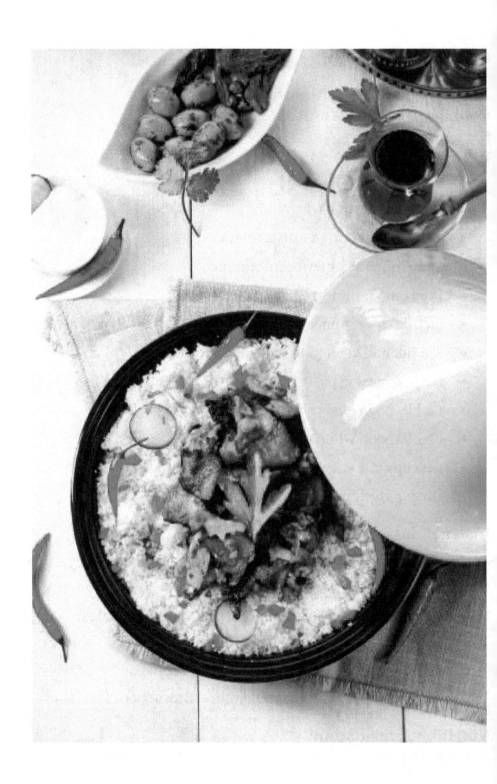

Dinner

Moroccan stir fry

Preparation time: 10 minutes
Cooking time: 20 minutes
Total time: 30 minutes
Serves: 2
Ingredients

- ¼ cup onion
- 1 clove garlic
- 1 lb. Ground salmon
- 1 tsp all spice
- 1 tsp cumin
- 1 tsp salt
- 2 cups cabbage
- 1 tablespoon mint
- 1 red bell pepper
- Zest of 1 lemon
- 1 tablespoon lemon juice
- Plain yogurt
- Pint leaves

Instructions

1. In a skillet heat olive oil and sauté garlic, onion until soft
2. Add cumin, pepper, salt, all spice, ground salmon and sauté for 8-10 minutes
3. Add cabbage, red bell pepper, pint leaves, lemon zest and sauté for 4-5 minutes
4. When ready garnish with mint leaves, yogurt and serve

Asian kebabs

Preparation time: 10 minutes
Cooking time: 20 minutes
Total time: 30 minutes
Serves: 8-12
Ingredients

- 2 lb. Tuna
- 8-10 skewers
- Romain lettuce leaves
- Green onions

Marinade

- ¼ cup coconut aminos
- 1 tablespoon water
- 1 tablespoon olive oil
- 2 cloves garlic
- 2 cloves onions
- 1 tablespoon sesame seeds
- 1 tsp pepper flakes

Instructions

1. Place all ingredients for the marinade in a bowl and mix well
2. place tuna cubes into the marinade bowl and let the meat marinade at least 8 hours
3. Preheat grill and place the tuna kebabs on the grill
4. Cook for 4-5 minutes per side
5. When ready remove the kebabs from the gill and serve on lettuce leaves with green onions

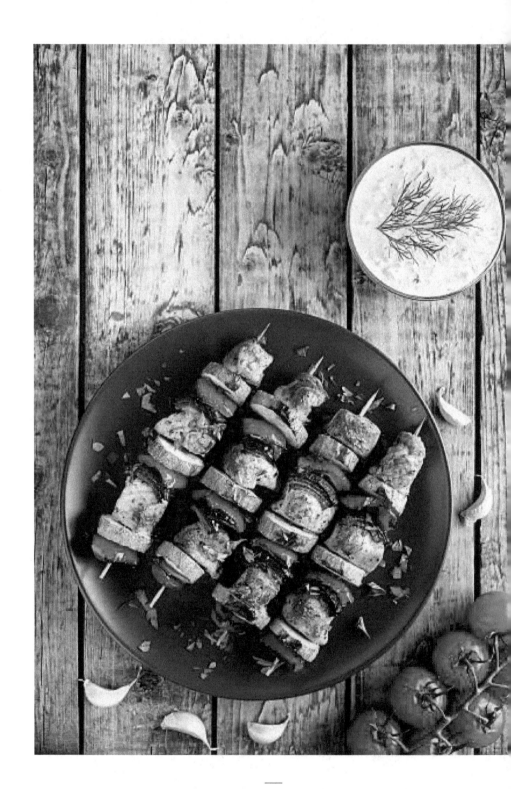

Chickpea stew

Preparation time: 15 minutes

Cooking time: 45 minutes

Total time: 60 minutes

Serves: 4

Ingredients

- 2 garlic cloves
- 1 tablespoon olive oil
- 2 scallions
- 1 red bell pepper
- 1 tsp paprika
- 1 tsp cumin
- 3 cups chickpeas
- 3-4 mint leaves
- ½ cup white wine

Instructions

1. Chop all ingredients in big chunks
2. In a large pot heat olive oil and add ingredients one by one
3. Cook for 5-6 or until slightly brown
4. Add remaining ingredients and cook until tender, 35-45 minutes
5. Season while stirring on low heat
6. When ready remove from heat and serve

Butternut squash salad

Preparation time: 5 minutes

Cooking time: 5 minutes

Total time: 10 minutes

Serves: 2

Ingredients

- 3 cups butternut squash
- 1 cup cooked couscous
- 2 cups kale leaves
- 2 tablespoons cranberries
- 2 oz. Goat cheese
- 1 cup salad dressing

Instructions

1. In a bowl combine all ingredients together and mix well
2. Serve with dressing

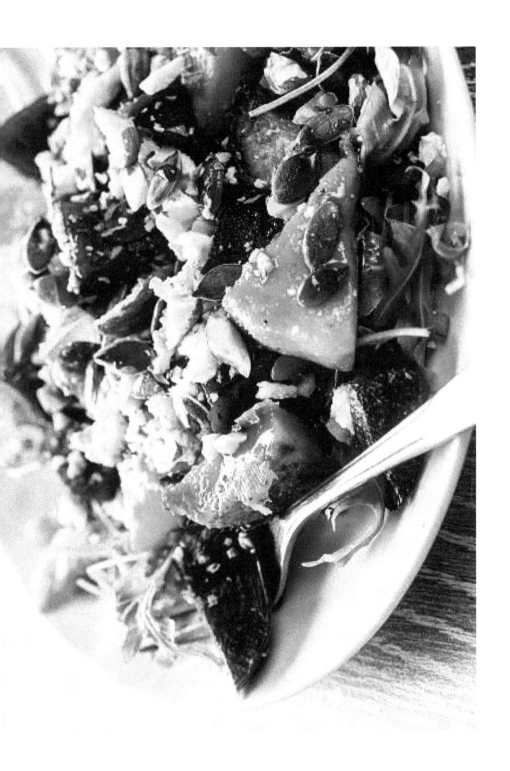

quinoa salad

Preparation time: 5 minutes

Cooking time: 5 minutes

Total time: 10 minutes

Serves: 2

Ingredients

- 1 cup cooked quinoa
- 1 tablespoon olive oil
- 1 tablespoon mustard
- 2 tablespoons lemon juice
- 1 cucumber
- ½ red onion
- ½ cup almonds
- 1 tablespoon mint

Instructions

1. In a bowl combine all ingredients together and mix well
2. Serve with dressing

Mediterranean budda bowl

Preparation time: 10 minutes

Cooking time: 10 minutes

Total time: 20 minutes

Serves: 1

Ingredients

- 1 zucchini
- ¼ tsp oregano
- Salt
- 1 cup cooked quinoa
- 1 cup spinach
- 1 cup mixed greens
- ½ cup red pepper
- ¼ cup cucumber
- ¼ cup tomatoes
- Parsley
- Tahini dressing

Instructions

1. In a skillet heat olive oil olive and sauté zucchini until soft and sprinkle oregano over zucchini
2. In a bowl add the rest of ingredients and toss to combine
3. Add fried zucchini and mix well
4. Pour over tahini dressing, mix well, and serve

Vegan curry

Preparation time: 10 minutes

Cooking time: 20 minutes

Total time: 30 minutes

Serves: 4

Ingredients

- 1 tablespoon olive oil
- ¼ cup onion
- 2 stalks celery
- 1 garlic clove
- ¼ tsp coriander
- ¼ tsp cumin
- ¼ tsp turmeric
- ¼ tsp red pepper flakes
- 1 cauliflower
- 1 zucchini
- 2 tomatoes
- 1 tsp salt
- 1 cup vegetable broth
- 1 handful of baby spinach
- 1 tablespoon almonds
- 1 tablespoon cilantro

Instructions

1. In a skillet heat olive oil and sauté celery, garlic, and onions for 4-5 minutes or until vegetables are tender

2. Add cumin, spices, coriander, cumin, turmeric red pepper flakes stir to combine and cook for another 1-2 minutes

3. Add zucchini, cauliflower, tomatoes, broth, spinach, water, and simmer on low heat for 15-20 minutes

4. Add remaining ingredients and simmer for another 4-5 minutes

5. Garnish curry and serve

Brussels sprouts

Preparation time: 10 minutes

Cooking time: 20 minutes

Total time: 30 minutes

Serves: 2

Ingredients

- 1 tablespoon olive oil
- 2 shallots
- 2 cloves garlic
- 1 lb. Brussels sprouts
- 1 cup vegetable stock
- 4 springs thyme
- ¼ cup pine nuts

Instructions

1. In a pan heat olive oil and cook shallots until tender
2. Add garlic, sprouts, thyme, stock and cook for another 4-5 minutes
3. Cover and cook for another 10-12 minutes or until sprouts are soft
4. When ready add pine nuts and serve

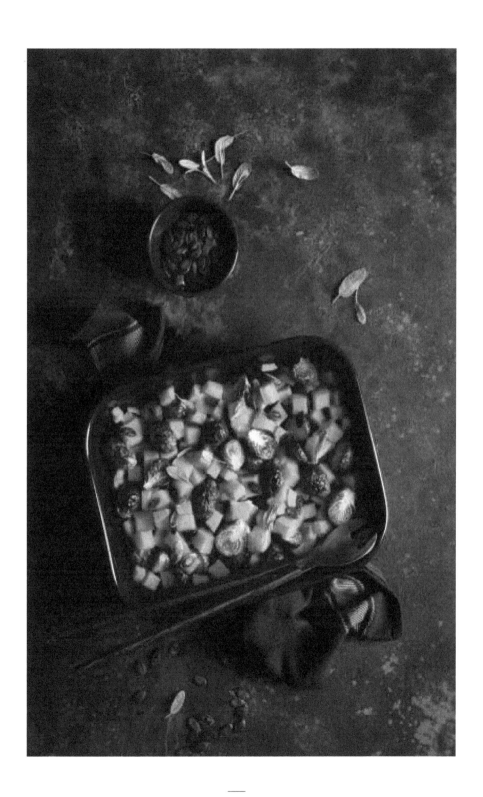

Entrée

Haddock Pie (Instant Pot)

Preparation Time: 10 minutes
Cooking Time: 15 Minutes
Serves: 3 Servings

Ingredients

- 1-pound haddock, cut into bite-sizes pieces
- 10 ounces frozen corns
- 10 ounces of frozen peas
- 1 teaspoon salt
- ½ teaspoon ground black pepper
- ¼ cup breadcrumbs
- ½ cup cream cheese
- 2/3 cup milk, unsweetened
- ½ cup cheddar cheese shredded

Instructions

1. Take a large bowl, pour in the milk, and then stir in cream cheese until well mixed.

2. Take another large bowl and place the haddock in it. Add corn and peas, and season with salt and black pepper. Then stir until combined.

3. Switch on the 4-quarts instant pot and scoop the haddock mixture in the inner pot and then add a layer with the prepared milk mixture.

4. Close the cover of the instant pot securely and press the manual button. Select the high-pressure setting, and then cook for 5 minutes. The instant pot will take 5 to 10 minutes to build pressure, by then, the cooking timer will start.

5. Meanwhile, switch on the oven, then set it up to 140 degrees F and preheat.

6. In a medium bowl, place breadcrumbs in it. Add cheese, and then stir until mixed.

7. When the instant pot beeps, let the pressure release naturally and then carefully open the instant pot.

8. Scoop the haddock mixture into a pie dish. Top with cheddar-breadcrumbs mixture, then bake for 10 minutes until the top turns golden brown.

9. When done, let the pie rest for 5 minutes and then serve.

Nutrition Information

Carbohydrates: 48.8 grams; Fat: 32.2 grams; Protein: 26.6 grams; Fiber: 7.2 grams; Calories: 591.7

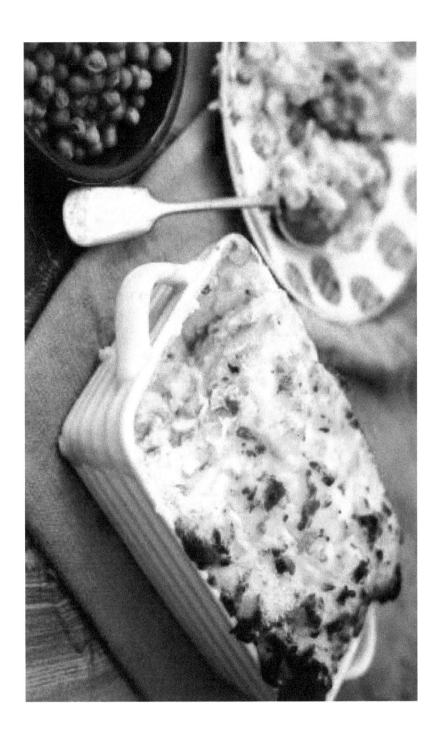

Panko Crusted Fried Haddock (Air Fryer)

Preparation Time: 5 minutes

Cooking Time: 24 Minutes

Serves: 4 Servings (1 fillet per serving)

Ingredients

- 4 fillets of haddock fish, each about 5 ounces
- ½ cup all-purpose flour
- 1 teaspoon salt
- ½ teaspoon ground black pepper
- 6 tablespoons mayonnaise
- 2 eggs
- 3 cups panko breadcrumbs

Instructions

1. Place salt and black pepper in a shallow dish. Add panko breadcrumbs, and then stir until mixed.
2. Use another shallow dish and place the flour in it.
3. Crack the eggs in another shallow dish, add mayonnaise and then whisk until blended.
4. Switch on the air fryer and grease the fryer's basket with oil. Insert it into the fryer and close the cover. Select the cooking temperature up to 350 degrees F and preheat.
5. Work on one fish fillet at a time, dredge into the flour mixture. Dip into the mayonnaise mixture, and then lightly coat into breadcrumbs mixture.
6. Arrange the prepared fish fillets in a single layer, and place into the fryer's basket. Spray with oil. Close the cover, and cook for 12 minutes until golden brown, and crisp, turning halfway through and spraying with oil.
7. Serve right away.

Nutrition Information

Carbohydrates: 33.7 grams; Fat: 21 grams; Protein: 43.7 grams; Fiber: 1.5 grams; Calories: 500

Lemon Pepper Haddock (Air Fryer)

Preparation Time: 10 minutes

Cooking Time: 12 Minutes

Serves: 1 Serving (1 fillet per serving)

Ingredients

- 1 fillet of haddock, about 8 ounces
- 1/3 cup panko breadcrumbs
- ¼ cup all-purpose flour
- 2 teaspoons lemon pepper seasoning
- 2 egg whites
- 2 slices of lemon
- 2 tablespoons chopped parsley

Instructions

1. Switch on the air fryer and grease the fryer's basket with oil. Insert it into the fryer and close the cover. Select the cooking temperature up to 350 degrees F and preheat.

2. Get a shallow dish, and place flour in it.

3. Use another shallow dish, and place egg whites. Then whisk until blended.

4. Add breadcrumbs, and lemon pepper seasoning in a shallow dish, then stir until mixed.

5. First, lightly coat the fish into the flour. Dip into the egg, and then coat the fish into the breadcrumbs 'mixture, pressing into the fish.

6. Place the prepared fish into the fryer's basket, and spray with oil. Close the cover, and then cook for 12 minutes until golden brown and crisp, turning halfway, and spraying with oil.

7. When done, garnish with parsley and serve the fish with lemon slices.

Nutrition Information

Carbohydrates: 47 grams; Fat: 1.3 grams; Protein: 51.1 grams; Fiber: 3 grams; Calories: 409

Caribbean Fried Smoked Herring (Pan)

Preparation Time: 10 minutes

Cooking Time: 15 Minutes

Serves: 3 Servings

Ingredients

- 8 ounces smoked herring fillets
- ½ cup diced white onions
- 1 hot pepper, minced
- ½ cup diced tomatoes
- 2 green onions, thinly sliced, white and green parts separated
- ½ teaspoon minced garlic
- 2 tablespoons olive oil
- 1 tablespoon minced thyme
- ½ tablespoon lemon juice
- Water as needed

Instructions

1. Use a medium saucepan, place it over medium-high heat. Add herring fillets, and then cover with water.

2. Bring to a boil. Let the fish boil for 5 minutes, then drain the water completely and set aside until needed.

3. Let the fish cool slightly, and then chop into small pieces, and set aside.

4. Get a large skillet pan, place it over medium heat, and add oil.

5. Add onion, toss until coated in oil. Then cook for 5 minutes until onions have turned tender.

6. Add garlic, tomatoes, thyme, and hot pepper. Stir until mixed, and then continue cooking for 1 minute.

7. Add the drained herring into the pan and toss until well mixed. Cook for 5 minutes, and then stir in green onions, and lemon juice.

8. Remove the pan from heat and serve immediately.

Nutrition Information

Carbohydrates: 21 grams; Fat: 25 grams; Protein: 12 grams; Fiber: 3 grams; Calories: 348

Fried Herring (Air Fryer)

Preparation Time: 10 minutes
Cooking Time: 20 Minutes
Serves: 4 Servings (1 fish per serving)
Ingredients

- 5 herrings, scaled, gutted, cleaned, rinsed
- 5 tablespoons pastry flour or all-purpose flour
- 2 teaspoons salt
- 2 teaspoons ground black pepper
- ½ cup chopped parsley
- 1 lemon, cut into wedges
- Non-stick cooking oil spray

Instructions

1. Switch on the air fryer and grease the fryer's basket with oil. Insert it into the fryer and close the cover. Select the cooking temperature up to 400 degrees F and preheat.
2. Prepare the herring. Remove the scales, its insides, and then rinse well.
3. Season the herring with salt, and black pepper, then coat it with flour.
4. Arrange the prepared herring in a single layer into the fryer' basket, and spray with oil. Close the cover, and then cook for 10 minutes until golden brown and crisp, turning halfway, and spraying with oil.
5. When done, transfer fried herring to a plate. Garnish with parsley, and then serve with lemon wedges.

Nutrition Information

Carbohydrates: 10.9 grams; Fat: 9.4 grams; Protein: 37 grams; Fiber: 0.9 grams; Calories: 276

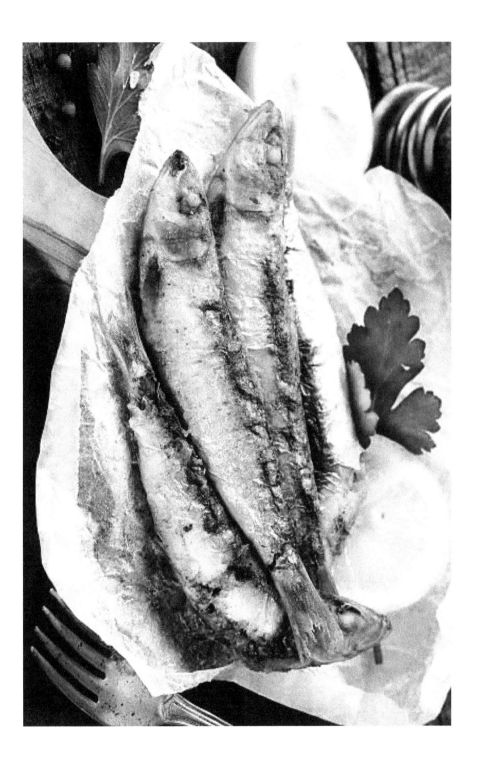

Smoked Salmon and Herring on Toasted Baguette (Oven)

Preparation Time: 10 minutes

Cooking Time: 10 Minutes

Serves: 6 Servings (2 toasts per serving)

Ingredients

- 7 ounces smoked salmon
- 1 teaspoon salt
- 3 ounces canned herring fillets, chopped
- ½ teaspoon dried thyme
- ½ teaspoon dried parsley
- ½ teaspoon ground black pepper
- ½ teaspoon dried rosemary
- 1 tablespoon lemon zest
- 1 tablespoon chopped fresh dill
- 2 tablespoons lemon juice
- 1 ciabatta baguette
- 2 tablespoons olive oil

Instructions

1. Switch on the oven and set it up to 400 degrees F and preheat.
2. Meanwhile, cut the baguette in half (lengthwise), and brush the inside with oil. Then sprinkle it with salt.
3. Place the cut baguettes into the oven. Bake for 5 minutes, or more until slightly toasted.
4. When done, sprinkle thyme, parsley, black pepper, and rosemary on the baguettes. Cut each baguette into six slices.
5. Top each baguette slice with herring and salmon. Sprinkle lemon zest and dill on top, and then drizzle with lemon juice.
6. Serve right away.

Nutrition Information

Carbohydrates: 15.1 grams; Fat: 7.9 grams; Protein: 11.5 grams; Fiber: 0.7 grams; Calories: 178

Lobster Tails (Instant Pot)

Preparation Time: 10 minutes

Cooking Time: 1 Minutes

Serves: 2 Servings (1 lobster tail per serving)

Ingredients

- 2 lobster tails
- 1 teaspoon of sea salt
- 1 teaspoon garlic powder
- ½ teaspoon ground white pepper
- 1 teaspoon smoked paprika
- 1 ½ tablespoon butter, unsalted, divided
- 1 cup of water
- ¼ cup melted butter, unsalted

Instructions

1. Switch on the 4-quarts instant pot and fill the inner pot with water. Insert a trivet stand.
2. Place a lobster tail on a baking sheet, and then cut the top of the tail shell down to its tip with kitchen scissors.
3. Remove any grit or vein from the lobster tail. Pull the shell down so that meat looks on top of crab shell. Slide a lemon wedge between the lobster's tail and meat. Do the same with the other lobster tail.
4. Place salt in a small bowl. Add garlic powder, white pepper, and paprika. Stir until well mixed, and then sprinkle mixture on the meat.
5. Top the meat with small pieces of butter and arrange the crabs' tails on the trivet stand. Close the cover of the instant pot securely.
6. Press the manual button, sand elect the high-pressure setting. Cook for 1 minute. The instant pot will take 5 to 10 minutes to build pressure, and then the cooking timer will start.
7. When the instant pot beeps, quickly release the pressure, and open the instant pot. Let the lobster tail rest in the instant pot for 10 minutes.
8. Place the lobster tail to a serving dish and then serve with melted butter.

Nutrition Information

Carbohydrates: 0.7 grams; Fat: 24 grams; Protein: 21 grams; Fiber: 0 grams; Calories: 301

Lobster Risotto (Instant Pot)

Preparation Time: 5 minutes

Cooking Time: 25 Minutes

Serves: 2 Servings (1 bowl per serving)

Ingredients

- 1 cup Arborio rice, rinsed
- 2 lobster tails, each about 4 ounces
- 1 large shallot, peeled, minced
- 1 ½ teaspoon minced garlic
- 1 leek, sliced
- ¾ teaspoon salt
- 1/3 teaspoon ground black pepper
- 1 tablespoon chopped thyme leaves
- 1 tablespoon butter, unsalted
- 1 tablespoon olive oil
- ½ cup brandy
- 3 tablespoon mascarpone cheese
- 2 cups fish stock
- 1 tablespoon chopped thyme leaves

Instructions

1. Fill a large pot with a half full salted water. Place it over medium-high heat and bring to a boil.
2. Add lobster tails, boil for 7 minutes, or more until the tails curl and turn bright red in color. Then, drain the remaining water.
3. Let the lobster tails cool for 10 minutes, cut them open by cutting lengthwise along the back of the shell. Use a kitchen shear, and then chop the lobsters' meat. Set aside until needed.
4. Switch on the 4-quarts instant pot and press the sauté button.
5. Add butter and oil into the inner pot and let the butter melts. Add shallots and leeks, and then cook for 2 minutes until vegetables begin to soften.
6. Add garlic and stir until well mixed. Cook for 1 minute, then add rice. Stir until well combined.
7. Pour brandy into the inner pot and bring it to a simmer. Pour in the fish stock and stir until well blended. Press the cancel button.
8. Close the cover of the instant pot securely. Press the manual button and select the high-pressure setting. Cook for 6 minutes. The instant pot will take 5 to 10 minutes to build pressure, and then the cooking timer will start.
9. When the instant pot beeps, quickly release the pressure, and then open the instant pot carefully.
10. Add salt, black pepper, and cheese into the risotto. Stir until cheese melts, and then place evenly in two bowls.
11. Top the risotto with lobsters' meat, and garnish with thyme, then serve.

Nutrition Information

Carbohydrates: 43 grams; Fat: 8 grams; Protein: 21 grams; Fiber: 0 grams; Calories: 339

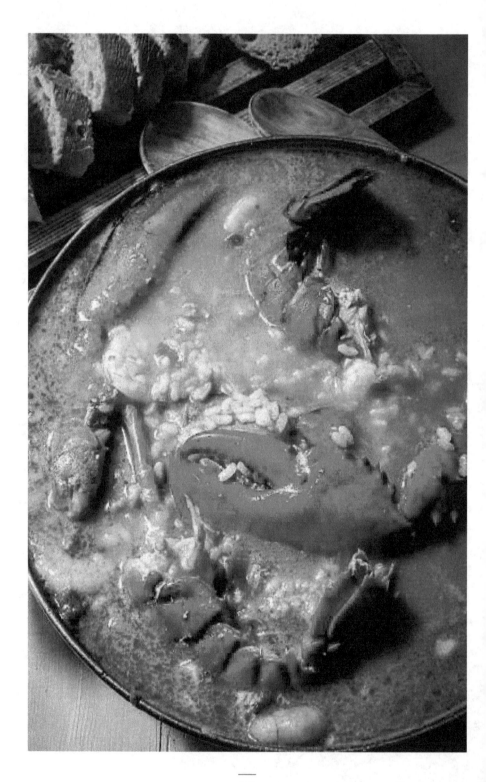

Lobster and Bacon Chowder (Instant Pot)

Preparation Time: 5 minutes
Cooking Time: 25 Minutes
Serves: 6 Servings (1 bowl per serving)

Ingredients

- 2 cups canned lobster meat
- 2 leeks, thinly sliced
- 3 cups frozen corn kernels
- 2 stalks of celery, diced
- 4 bacon slices, diced
- 2 medium red potatoes, unpeeled, diced
- 1 teaspoon salt
- 1 tablespoon corn starch
- ½ teaspoon ground black pepper
- 1 cup heavy cream
- 4 cups lobster stock or chicken broth
- 2 tablespoons chopped chives

Instructions

1. Switch on the 4-quarts instant pot and press the sauté button. Preheat until hot.
2. Add bacon slices and cook for 5 minutes until crisp. Transfer bacon to a plate, and reserve 1 tablespoon of bacon fat from the inner pot.
3. Add leeks, and celery into the inner pot. Cook for 3 minutes until vegetables become soft and press the cancel button.
4. Return cooked bacon into the inner pot and add corn and potatoes. Pour in the stock and stir until well combined.
5. Close the cover of the instant pot securely. Press the manual button and select the high-pressure setting. Cook for 7 minutes. The instant pot will take 5 to 10 minutes to build pressure, and then the cooking timer will start.
6. Meanwhile, using a small bowl, add cream, and whisk in cornstarch until well combined.
7. When the instant pot beeps, quickly release pressure, and then carefully open the instant pot.
8. Press the sauté button and add the cream mixture. Stir for 1 minute and bring the chowder to a simmer. Cook for 1 to 2 minutes until chowder has thickened.
9. Add lobster meat and stir until mixed. Simmer for 3 to 4 minutes until thoroughly hot, and then press the cancel button.
10. Season the chowder with salt and black pepper. Garnish with chives, and then serve.

Nutrition Information

Carbohydrates: 20.1 grams; Fat: 13.1 grams; Protein: 11.3 grams; Fiber: 2 grams; Calories: 236.5

Smoothie

Ginger Colada Smoothie

Preparation time: 5 minutes

Cooking time: 5 minutes

Total time: 10 minutes

Serves: 1

Ingredients

- 1 tablespoon ginger
- ½ cup lemon juice
- 1 cup pineapple
- 1 banana
- 1 handful spinach
- 1 handful kale
- 1 cup ice

Instructions

1. In a blender place all ingredients and blend until smooth
2. Pour smoothie in a glass and serve

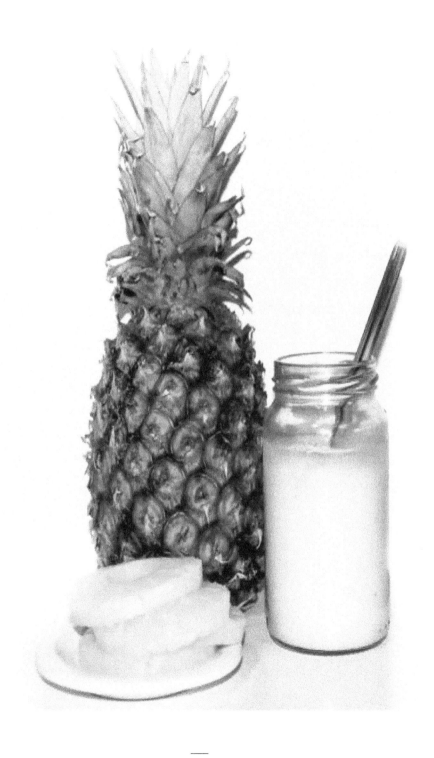

Acai Smoothie

Preparation time: 5 minutes

Cooking time: 5 minutes

Total time: 10 minutes

Serves: 1

Ingredients

- 1 cup acai puree
- 1 banana
- 1 cup pomegranate juice
- 1 kiwi
- ½ lemon

Instructions

1. In a blender place all ingredients and blend until smooth
2. Pour smoothie in a glass and serve

Soy Smoothie

Preparation Time: 5 Minutes

Cooking Time: 5 Minutes

Total Time: 10 Minutes

Serves: 1

Ingredients

- 2 cups blueberries
- 1 cup soy vanilla yogurt
- 1 cup soy milk
- 1 tsp vanilla essence

Instructions

1. In a blender place all ingredients and blend until smooth
2. Pour smoothie in a glass and serve

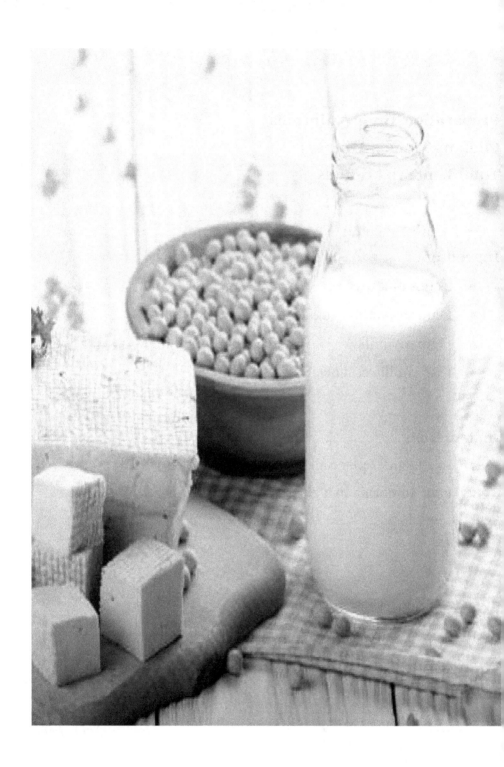

Oat Smoothie

Preparation Time: 5 Minutes
Cooking Time: 5 Minutes
Total Time: 10 Minutes
Serves: 1

Ingredients

- 1 cup orange juice
- ¼ cup oats
- 1 tablespoon flaxseed meal
- 1 tablespoon honey
- 1 banana
- 1 cup ice

Instructions

1. In a blender place all ingredients and blend until smooth
2. Pour smoothie in a glass and serve

Chocolate Oat Smoothie

Preparation Time: 10 Minutes

Cooking Time: 0 minutes

Servings: 2

Ingredients

- ½ cup rolled oats
- 3 tablespoon cocoa powder, unsweetened
- 2 teaspoon flax seeds
- 2 large frozen bananas
- ¼ teaspoon sea salt
- ¼ teaspoon cinnamon
- ½ teaspoon vanilla extract, unsweetened
- 4 tablespoons almond butter
- 2 cup coconut milk, unsweetened

Instructions

1. Place all the ingredients in the order in a food processor or blender and then pulse for 2 to 3 minutes at high speed until smooth.
2. Pour the smoothie into a glass and then serve.

Nutrition Information

Calories: 262; Fat: 7g; Protein: 8g; Carbohydrates: 50g

Fruity Tofu Smoothie

Preparation Time: 10 Minutes

Cooking Time: 0 Minutes

Servings: 2

Ingredients

- 12 ounces silken tofu, pressed and drained
- 2 medium bananas, peeled
- 1½ cups fresh blueberries
- 1 tablespoon maple syrup
- 1½ cups unsweetened soymilk
- ¼ cup ice cubes

Instructions

1. Place all the ingredients in a high-speed blender and pulse until creamy.
2. Pour into two glasses and serve immediately.

Nutrition Information

Calories: 398; Total fat: 8g; Carbohydrates: 65g; Protein: 20g

Green Fruity Smoothie

Preparation Time: 10 Minutes

Cooking Time: 0 Minutes

Servings: 2

Ingredients

- 1 cup frozen mango, peeled, pitted, and chopped
- 1 large frozen banana, peeled
- 2 cups fresh baby spinach
- 1 scoop unsweetened vegan vanilla protein powder
- ¼ cup pumpkin seeds
- 2 tablespoons hemp hearts
- 1½ cups unsweetened almond milk

Instructions

1. In a high-speed blender, place all the ingredients and pulse until creamy.
2. Pour into two glasses and serve immediately.

Nutrition Information

Calories: 355; Total fat: 16g; Carbohydrates: 35g; Protein: 23g

Pineapple Coconut Chia Smoothie

Preparation Time: 10 Minutes
Cooking Time: 0 Minutes
Servings: 2

Ingredients

- 2 cup Coconut Milk
- 2 cup Pineapple, frozen
- 1 Ginger Piece
- 1 cup Kale, stems discarded
- 2 tsp. Chia Seeds
- 2/3 cup Mint Leaves
- 1 cup Spinach Leaves
- 2 Lime, peel & rind removed

Instructions

1. To start, place all the ingredients into a high-speed blender and blend for a minute or two or until you get a smooth drink.
2. Serve immediately and enjoy.

Nutrition Information

Calories: 313; Protein: 35g; Carbohydrates: 30g; Fats: 9g

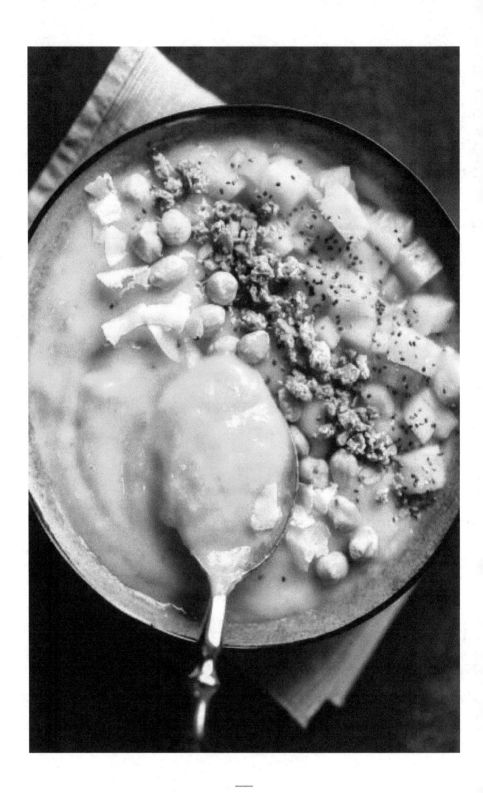

Specials

Amaranth "Risotto" With Mushrooms

Preparation Time: 10 Minutes

Cooking Time: 50 minutes

Servings: 2

Ingredients

- 1-ounce dried porcini mushrooms (about 1 cup)
- 2 cups boiling water plus 2 1/2 cups cold water
- 6 tablespoons unsalted butter
- 2 tablespoons olive oil
- 1 large yellow onion, finely chopped (about 1 1/2 cups)
- 2 cups amaranth
- 1 1/2 teaspoons salt, or to taste
- 3 garlic cloves, finely chopped
- 1-pound sliced mushrooms (white, baby Bella, cremini, or a mixture)
- 1 tablespoon soy sauce
- 3 tablespoons sherry (any type from dry to cream)
- Freshly ground black pepper to taste
- 1 teaspoon chopped fresh thyme, or to taste

Instructions

1. Put 2 cups boiling water on dried porcini mushrooms in heatproof bowl: soak porcini mushrooms for 10-15 minutes till tender. Lift from liquid; squeeze extra liquid into bowl.
2. Chop porcini mushrooms finely. Separately reserve liquid and porcini mushrooms. Warm 1 tbsp. oil and 1 tbsp. butter in 4-qt. heavy pot on medium low heat. Add onion; cook, covered, occasionally mixing, for 10-15 minutes till lightly golden and tender.
3. Add amaranth; mix to coat in oil and butter. Add reserved porcini mushroom soaking liquid slowly; leave grit at bottom of bowl.
4. Add 2 1/2 cups cold water then cover pot: boil, occasionally whisking. Push seeds clinging to side of pot into liquid with heatproof rubber spatula.
5. Lower heat to low; simmer, covered, for 20-25 minutes till liquid is absorbed.
6. Mix in 1 tsp. (or to taste) salt. Take off heat; stand for 5-10 minutes, covered.
7. As amaranth simmers, melt 1 tbsp. leftover oil and 1 tbsp. leftover butter in 12-in. heavy skillet on medium heat.
8. Add garlic; cook for 30 seconds, mixing.
9. Add soy sauce, leftover 1/2 tsp. salt, reserved porcini mushrooms and fresh sliced mushrooms; sauté for 8-10 minutes till mushrooms are juicy and soft.
10. Add sherry; sauté for 2 minutes till mushrooms are tender.
11. Season with freshly ground black pepper and salt. Take off heat; mix in thyme.
12. Cut leftover 4 tbsp. butter to small pieces then add to pan; mix till melted. Put amaranth into soup bowls/onto plates.
13. Top with mushroom mixture

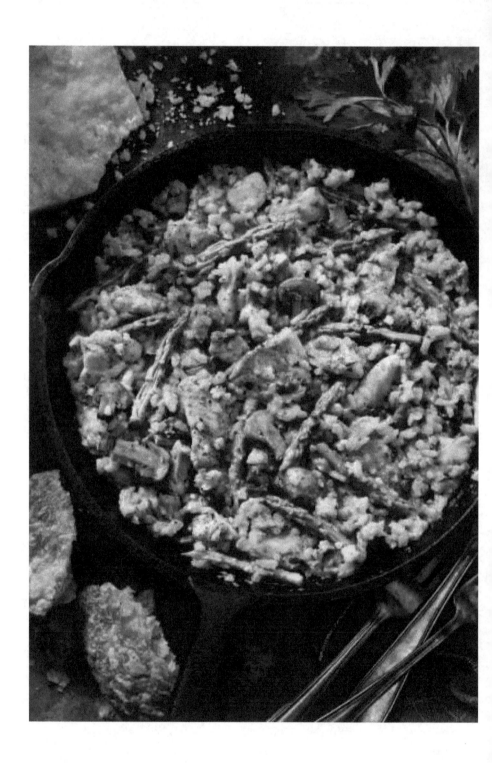

Asian Pear and Frisée Salad

Preparation Time: 10 Minutes
Cooking Time: 10 minutes
Servings: 2

Ingredients

- 1/2 cup balsamic vinegar
- 1 teaspoon packed brown sugar
- 2 medium leeks (white and pale green parts only), halved lengthwise and thinly sliced
- 1/4 cup extra-virgin olive oil
- 1/2-pound frisée, torn (8 cups)
- 1 large Asian pear (8 to 10 ounces), thinly sliced

Instructions

1. In a small heavy saucepan, boil the sugar, vinegar, and 1/4 tsp. of salt for 3 minutes, stirring until the mixture is reduced by half. Pour the mixture into a cup.
2. Rinse the leeks and pat them until dry. Cook the leeks in a cleaned saucepan with oil and 1/4 tsp. of salt over medium heat for 5 minutes, stirring for some time until softened.
3. Decorate the plates with pear and frisée and drizzle with hot leeks in oil, and then followed by the reduced vinegar.
4. Grind the pepper all over the salad.

Balsamic Mixed Vegetable Roast

Preparation Time: 30 Minutes

Cooking Time: 20 minutes

Servings: 4

Ingredients

- 2 medium eggplants, unpeeled, cut crosswise into 1/4-inch-thick rounds
- 2 teaspoons of salt, divided in half
- 1 cup extra-virgin olive oil
- 1/3 cup balsamic vinegar
- 1/2 teaspoon freshly ground black pepper
- 1 1/2 pounds zucchini, washed, dried, and cut on the bias into 1/4-inch rounds
- 3 large red onions, sliced into 1/4-inch rounds
- 2 medium red bell peppers, cored, seeded, and cut into 3/4-inch squares
- 2 medium yellow bell peppers, cored, seeded, and cut into 3/4-inch squares
- 6 large heads of endive, cored, halved, and quartered lengthwise
- Garnish: 4 sprigs fresh basil

Instructions

1. Put a layer of paper towels onto baking sheet. Place eggplant in single layers and drizzle in one teaspoon of salt. Allow to sit for half an hour. Pat dry.

2. Preheat an oven to 450°F.

3. Whisk pepper, remaining salt, vinegar, and olive oil together. Reserve.

4. Divide the endive, peppers, red onions, zucchini, and eggplant among two large baking pans with sides. Gently mix the veggies with vinegar and 3/4 of blended oil.

5. Put one baking sheet at the bottom rack of oven and another on the center rack. Roast the veggies for about 15 to 20 minutes, flipping them once and switching pans between the shelves after ten minutes. The veggies will be crisp when done.

6. Place the veggies in colorful bunches onto oval or round platters and combine the different types of vegetables together. Drizzle pepper and salt onto the vegetables. Then sprinkle with remaining olive oil/balsamic vinegar dressing. You can serve at room temperature.

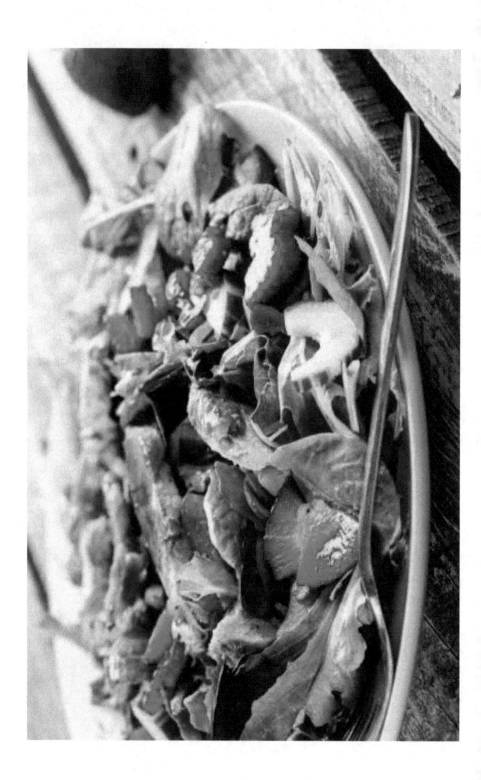

Basic Cake Doughnuts

Preparation Time: 20 Minutes

Cooking Time: 10 minutes

Servings: 4

Ingredients

- 3/4 cups (240 grams) all-purpose flour, sifted
- 2 teaspoons baking powder
- 1/2 teaspoon salt
- 1 teaspoon freshly grated nutmeg
- 1/3 cup (75 grams) superfine sugar
- 2 tablespoons (1 ounce) unsalted butter or vegetable shortening
- 1 egg
- 1/2 cup whole milk, scalded and divided
- 2 tablespoons plain yogurt
- 1 teaspoon vanilla extract
- Vegetable oil for frying

Instructions

1. Mix sugar, nutmeg, salt, baking powder and flour in a stand mixer bowl fastened with paddle attachment. Mix on low speed. Put in butter and mix at medium-low speed. Mixture must look much like coarse sand. Mix vanilla, yogurt, 1/4 cup milk and egg in another bowl.

2. Into the flour-butter mixture, gradually put wet ingredients while mixer is running.

3. Scrape down sides of bowl and stir for 20 seconds. Stir in the rest of the milk, a small amount at one time, till batter adheres to bowl sides. Batter must be spoonable, thick, smooth, and resembles moist cookie dough. You may not use all of the milk.

4. Put on plastic wrap to cover and allow to sit for 15 to 20 minutes.

5. In a heavy-based pot, heat at least 2 inches of oil till a deep-fat thermometer reads 360°F.

6. For traditional doughnuts, fill one piping bag fitted with 1/3-inch circle tip. Estimate the number of 3-inch doughnuts your pot can fry at a time. Oil a square 4×4-inch parchment square for each and onto every square, pipe a 3-inch diameter ring.

7. In the oil, carefully put one, parchment side facing up. Take the parchment out using tongs and do the same with several additional rings, being cautious not to overcrowd the pan.

8. Cook till light golden brown for 1 to 2 minutes per side. For the drop doughnuts, right into the oil, simply drop tablespoon-size dollops and fry till light golden brown for 45 seconds on each side.

9. Take them out using slotted spoon and put on paper towel to drain.

10. Do the same with the rest of the batter. Allow to cool just slightly prior to glazing and eating.

Berry Scones

Preparation Time: 10 Minutes

Cooking Time: 20 minutes

Servings: 4

Ingredients

- 2 cups all-purpose gluten-free flour
- 1 teaspoon xanthan gum
- 1 tablespoon baking powder
- 1/2 teaspoon kosher salt
- 2 tablespoons sugar
- 1 cup frozen berries (I love cranberries or blueberries here)
- 5 tablespoons unsalted butter, diced and chilled
- 1 cup milk (low-fat is fine, nonfat is not)

Instructions

1. Preheat oven to 400°F. Line parchment paper on baking sheets; put aside.

2. Mix sugar, salt, baking powder, xanthan gum and flour in a big bowl; put few tbsp. of dry ingredient mixture into small bowl.

3. Add frozen berries; toss till berries are coated. Put small bowl aside.

4. Add diced butter to big bowl with dry ingredients; cut it in till butter looks like pea-sized chunks covered with flour. You can use 2 knifes or a pastry cutter to do this then act like you are cutting steak again and again.

5. Put milk in butter/dry ingredient mixture; stir to mix. Dough should come together. Add berries to dough when dough comes together; gently fold in till they are distributed evenly throughout.

6. Turn dough onto lightly floured surface, handling as little as you can to avoid melting butter in your hands; pat to 1/2-in. thick rectangle.

7. Cut dough to 8 triangles; put triangles on parchment paper-lined baking sheets, few inches apart.

8. Brush bit of milk; if desired, sprinkle a bit of sugar.

9. Bake till scones slightly brown around edges and puffed up for 15-20 minutes; immediately serve.

Black and White Pancake Cake

Preparation Time: 10 Minutes + chilling time
Cooking Time: 50 minutes
Servings: 4

Ingredients

- 1 batch of Maple Chocolate Cake batter
- 1/2 cup (4 ounces/113 grams) water
- 1/2 cup (4 1/4 ounces/120 grams) heavy cream, chilled
- 1/2 cup (4 ounces/113 grams) mascarpone cheese, at room temperature
- 1 1/2 tablespoons (1 1/8 ounces/32 grams) pure maple syrup (dark or very dark preferred) *
- 1 teaspoon vanilla bean paste or pure vanilla extract
- 5 ounces (142 grams) bittersweet chocolate (60% to 70% cacao), chopped
- 6 tablespoons (3 ounces/85 grams) heavy cream
- A cast-iron griddle, about 10 × 17 inches in size**
- A very thin, flexible metal spatula, such as a fish spatula

Instructions

1. Preheat griddle for 10 minutes on low heat; should be hot on lowest heat possible to prevent burning pancakes and give enough time for them to cook through.
2. Pancakes: Make Maple Chocolate cake batch, adding water to wet ingredients then whisk batter till smooth.
3. Spray nonstick spray on griddle generously. 2 pancakes at 1 time, put 2 1/2-cup batter scoops onto griddle and swirl gently and coat pancakes to 7-in. circles with back of a spoon.
4. Cook pancakes for 4 minutes on 1st side till bubbles are not popping on surfaces and edges look dry.
5. Gently flip pancakes with a flexible, thin metal spatula; cook till centers of cake spring back when touched lightly for 2 minutes.
6. Transfer layers to wire racks; fully cool.
7. Repeat batter scooping then cooking process till you get 8 cake layers. Line parchment paper on 2 big baking sheets; on each sheet, put 4 cake layers in 1 layer. Chill for 10-15 minutes in the fridge.
8. Cream filling: Whip cream to stiff peaks on high speed in a medium bowl. Beat vanilla bean pasta, maple syrup and mascarpone on low speed for 30 seconds till it starts to thicken and is smooth in another medium bowl; do not overbeat. Mascarpone might seize.
9. Fold in whipped cream gently till smooth. Ganache filling: Mix cream and bittersweet chocolate in small heatproof bowl; microwave for 45-60 seconds on high power; whisk ganache till it has chocolate pudding texture, is smooth and chocolate melts. Put 2 tbsp. ganache into small bowl; for garnish, put aside.
10. Cake assembly: Take pancake layers from fridge. Look at layers; for top layer, put aside the best looking one. Put 1 cake layer onto cake stand/serving platter. Dollop 1/3 cup maple

mascarpone cream; smooth it out with small offset spatula, with 1/2-in. border all around.

11. Put 2nd layer over; to adhere, lightly press. Spread 2 1/2 tbsp. ganache onto layer with 1/2-in. border around cake. Repeat layer process 6 extra times, alternating chocolate ganache and mascarpone cream with layers; put best cake layer over.

Advice

To leftover chocolate ganache, add only around 1/2 tsp. drizzle cream to just thin out to honey-like consistency. If needed, warm ganache for 10 seconds to loosen up in microwave. Artfully drizzle ganache on cake; chill cake 30 minutes before serving. You can make cake 1 day ahead; 15 minutes before slicing, let soften on counter. Use darkest maple syrup in filling and cake to enhance flavor. You may use a heavy-bottomed very big skillet; just cook pancakes one by one.

Cooking time varies. If pancakes look like they will burn, lower heat accordingly like making regular pancakes (depends on your stove and griddle). Before cooking rest of layers, make small test pancake to test the heat.

Boxty

Preparation Time: 10 Minutes

Cooking Time: 60 minutes

Servings: 2

Ingredients

- 1/2-pound potatoes, unpeeled
- 1 1/2 cups buttermilk
- 1/2-pound potatoes, peeled and grated
- 1 3/4 cups all-purpose flour
- 1 teaspoon baking soda
- salt and ground black pepper to taste
- 2 tablespoons butter, or as needed

Instructions

1. Preheat oven to 450°F (230°C). Scrub the unpeeled potatoes and use a fork to prick them a few times; arrange onto a baking sheet.

2. In the preheated oven, bake 50 minutes to 1 hour until using a fork can easily pierce the potatoes. Remove from the oven, chill, and peel. Add buttermilk and mash with the potatoes.

3. Stir in pepper, salt, baking soda, flour and grated raw potato. In a large skillet or griddle, melt the butter over medium heat. Spoon into the skillet the potato mixture to make 3-inch cakes.

4. Fry about 5 minutes per side, turning once, until golden and crisp.

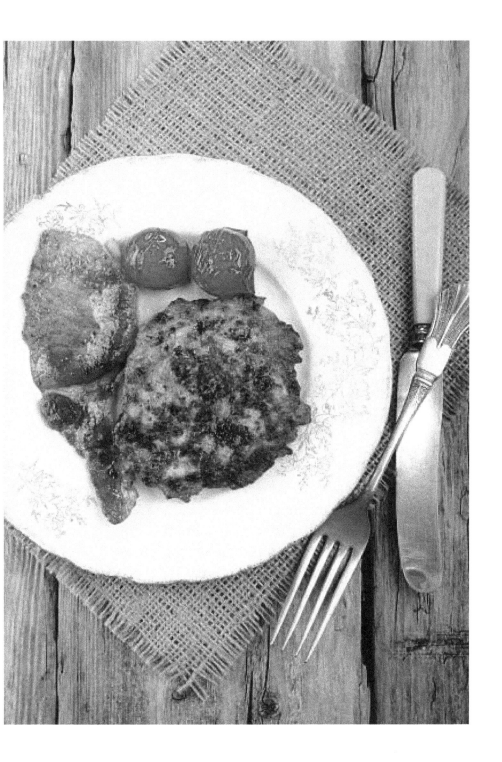

Bulgur Pilaf With Roasted Tomatoes, Onions, And Garbanzo Beans

Preparation Time: 10 Minutes
Cooking Time: 60 minutes
Servings: 2
Ingredients

- 2 pounds tomatoes, quartered
- 1 large onion, cut into 1/2-inch-thick wedges
- 2 tablespoons olive oil
- 1 15-ounce can garbanzo beans (chickpeas), drained
- 4 garlic cloves, crushed 2 1/2 cups water 2 cups bulgur* 4 tablespoons chopped fresh parsley
- 2 tablespoons chopped fresh dill
- 1 tablespoon fresh lemon juice

Instructions

1. Preheat the oven to 400 °F. In big roasting pan, scatter onion and tomatoes. Sprinkle oil over. Scatter with pepper and salt.
2. Roast for half an hour, mixing from time to time. Mix in garlic and garbanzo beans. Roast till onion turn golden, mixing from time to time, for an additional of 25 minutes.
3. Take pan out of oven. To pan, put 2 1/2 cups of water and mix, scratching up browned bits.
4. Turn mixture of roasted vegetable onto big saucepan. Boil.
5. Mix in bulgur. Lower the heat to low, put cover and let simmer for 10 minutes till bulgur is soft and liquid is soaked in.
6. Into pilaf, mix lemon juice, 1 1/2 tablespoons of dill and 3 tablespoons of parsley. Season with pepper and salt to taste.
7. Turn onto bowl. Scatter leftover one tablespoon of parsley and half tablespoon on dill on pilaf.

CPSIA information can be obtained
at www.ICGtesting.com
Printed in the USA
BVHW092314210621
610124BV00010B/1862